Ketogenic Diet for Rapid Weight Loss

Lose 30 Pounds in 30 Days

by FlatBelly Queens

Published in Great Britain by:

FlatBelly Queens
345 Old Street
London
EC1V 9LE

© Copyright 2016 – Flatbelly Queens

ISBN-13: {978-1533218094}
ISBN-10: {1533218099}

Table of Contents

INTRODUCTION

A way to lose weight quickly and keep it off is something that is on almost everybody's mind in this day and age. We are all looking for ways to slim down yet still eat delicious food. And we don't want to starve ourselves to get that beach body to feel healthier. After all, it is that constant feeling of hunger that causes most people to quit dieting. Or, you may have some health issues such as high blood pressure, heart disease, high cholesterol, or Type II diabetes and want to be able to control it through diet and possibly even be able to get off all those medications that you have to take to control it (yes, it is possible).

This book, the Ketogenic Diet for Rapid Weight Loss, is exactly what you are looking for! Billed as a high fat, low carbohydrate diet, many people the world over have found success losing weight and managing health issues through the use of the Ketogenic diet. This book will give you all the information that you need to begin following this diet. Reports have shown that people can start to lose weight fast, and can lose up to 30 pounds in 30 days when they stick to the program! You will look better, feel better, have more energy, and be able to face your life with the confidence that you have been looking for!

This book gives you all the information you need to get started on the road to weight loss and good health. The first chapter will define what the Ketogenic diet is, what it is not, and the mechanism for how it works to direct weight loss to the fat in your body, specifically the belly fat you carry around your midsection. This will then be followed by the history of the Ketogenic diet, from its earliest days to its multiple uses today. Many people don't realize that the Ketogenic diet was often used to control a variety of health issues, including epilepsy and diabetes, for hundreds of years! After that, this book will outline all the benefits of the Ketogenic diet, of which they are varied and vast. Following that is a chapter on the ten most frequently asked questions about the Ketogenic diet with their answers. Chapter five will then give you several tips and tricks to achieve the success you are going for on the Ketogenic diet. As you will learn, getting your body into the state of ketosis and staying in that state is the primary motivator to the fast weight loss on this diet. This last chapter will help you do just that, and by doing so, you will quickly achieve the results that you are looking for. There are several different things that you can do to maximize your success on the Ketogenic diet, and this chapter will discuss those things. The last section of this books is made up of Ketogenic recipes. This recipe section gives you seven breakfast, seven lunch, and seven dinner recipes to get you started on the Ketogenic diet.

It is important to note here that the Ketogenic diet is not just a weight loss fad. It has been used for thousands of years, as you will see in the history section. But, for this diet to work effectively, it should become a lifestyle, something that you incorporate into your life on a daily basis. Some people may think this is difficult, but once you realize how great it is to eat a high fat, low carb diet, you won't want to go back! There are so many wonderful recipes (many of them in this book) and limitless options for eating, you will soon find that you do not need carbs in your life! Once you have made this plan part of your life, you will see how much more energy you have, how good you will look and feel, and never want to go back to your old way of eating.

So let's get started. We begin with defining exactly what the Ketogenic diet is and what it can do for you.

Chapter 1: What is the Ketogenic Diet?

The easy definition of the Ketogenic diet is to eat low carbohydrate and high fat and adequate protein. It is often also called a low carb diet or a low carb high fat diet. The idea behind the diet is very simple: if you eat very few carbohydrates, your body will be forced to convert the stored fat in your body into energy because it does not have the more easily-burned carbohydrates to burn running through your system. A diet that is high in carbs, which is very typical for the average American person, gives the body a lot of easily digestible fuel.

Typically, the body uses carbohydrates ingested from food to fuel itself. Carbs are quickly and easily converted into simple sugars, which the body then uses for fuel. If you eat more calories than you can burn in a day, the body will then convert the fats and proteins you digest into fat that is stored throughout the body, usually in the belly, but also under the skin. Because your body is using the carbs for energy, the rest of the fuel you take in continues to be stored, leading to weight gain and belly fat.

However, if you move to a Ketogenic diet, you severely restrict the amount of carbohydrates you take in. Instead, you eat a diet that is high in fat, contains an adequate about of protein, with very few net carbs. The typical percentages for these macronutrients on the Ketogenic diet are 75 percent fats, 20 percent protein, and 5 percent net carbs. This forces your body to use something besides carbohydrates for fuel to get you through the day. Generally, your body will start to utilize the stored fat, converting it to energy that it can metabolize. This makes it very good for weight loss. Without the fast energy of carbohydrates to use, the body starts to burn its stores. This is great news for weight loss fans who are looking for a faster way to lose weight. Also, most of the fats burned comes from the dangerous "belly fat", the fat stored in your midsection, which is associated with higher levels of illness, diabetes, and heart disease.

This phase, where the body uses its own fat stores for energy, is called ketosis. It is so called because, as the body starts to break down its own stores of fat in the liver, ketones are produced through the process. These ketones are then used for energy by the body. To test whether your body is in a state of ketosis, you can use something called a Ketostix to test the urine to see if the body is, indeed, in a state of ketosis. The ketones will show up in your urine. Ketostix can generally be bought at any drug store or pharmacy. Although there is some debate about how accurate Ketostix are, they can be used as a good guide as to whether you are in this state and if, therefore, the diet will work as suggested.

To enter ketosis, you need to seriously reduce the amount of carbs that you take in through your diet. The fewer carbs you take in, the faster your body will enter the state of ketosis, and the sooner you will start to lose weight. Generally, most people who recommend a keto diet recommend taking in between 20 and 30 grams of net carbohydrates in a day, or about five percent of your daily caloric intake. A net carb is not the total amount of carbs. To define what a net carb is, you need to take the total amount of carbs in the food you eat minus the total fiber in that food. So, let us take the vegetable broccoli as an example. Broccoli has a total of 6 grams of carbohydrates in a cup, but 2 grams of that are of fiber. So, if you eat a cup of broccoli, your net carb total will be 4 grams. Fiber is still necessary in the diet and are not burned as easily as sugars in the digestive system, so they are still necessary for proper functioning of your body, including the bowels (which we will discuss later).

In general, the Ketogenic diet recommends that you eat 25 percent of your foods as proteins, 70 percent as fats, and only 5 percent of your food intake should be through carbohydrates. Any carbohydrates that you do eat should come from vegetables, nuts, and dairy. Refined carbs, such as wheat products, starch, or fruit, are to be avoided.

Remember, the Ketogenic diet is a lifestyle change. Once you have gotten into the diet and your body becomes used to it, you may find that you never want to stop eating this way! That is what we hope will happen. Once you see how good the food is and how you feel, you will never want to fill your body with carbs and sugars again.

The next chapter will discuss the history of the Ketogenic diet, and of low carb diets in general. It will also describe the differences between the different types of low carb diets.

CHAPTER 2:

The History of Keto

It is interesting to note that low carbohydrate, high fat diets may go back to the beginning of human history. It has been theorized that in Paleolithic days, humans only ate the meat that could be hunted or scavenged and foods that could be collected through gathering from the land. Before the advent of agriculture, humans ate very few carbohydrates, especially grains. Things such as wheat were not available to them. This was the diet that our bodies were evolved to eat. This is the theory behind why so many people have difficulties in eating the high carbohydrate diet that is so common today: our bodies and digestive systems have not evolved to eat this way and the body reacts badly to the carbs and sugars we are putting into ourselves. When people go back to a diet that is more like the one we evolved eating, the body functions better.

The use of the low carb, high fat ketogenic diet for the treatment of diabetes goes as far back as the year 1797 when it was used to control diabetes in two Army officers. It was the standard treatment for diabetes through the 1800s, before there were medicines available for treating diabetes. It was found to be a successful way to control the disease.

The modern start of the Ketogenic diet comes from one of the most unlikely places one would expect: it was created as a cure for epilepsy! As long ago as 500 BC, fasting was used to treat epilepsy. Somehow, not eating caused a decrease in the amount of seizures people had. After using fasting as a treatment for seizures, it was discovered that using a low carb, high fat diet was just as effective to preventing seizures as was fasting, without the pain of having to starve to get some relief. It was the perfect compromise between fasting and controlling seizures, and was used in many societies, including the Greeks. Modern medicine returned to using the practice of using the Ketogenic diet to treat childhood epilepsy in the 1920s. Although a small number of hospitals still utilize diet as a therapy for childhood epilepsy, the practice fell out of favor when anticonvulsive drugs were introduced. Until the advent of medications for seizures, the ketogenic diet was used effectively to treat epilepsy in children. More recently, with the backlash against the medical community, the Ketogenic diet is making a resurgence in its use as a treatment for seizure disorders because it does work. Plus, it can keep people off medications that have a great many side effects that are not a problem with controlling seizures through diet.

If you are wondering about the efficacy of using the Ketogenic diet for epilepsy, studies have shown that about half of the children treated with the ketogenic diet had their seizure numbers drop by at least half, and some had even greater success. The only real problem that these kids had on this diet was the risk of constipation. It was discovered that the history of constipation with following the Ketogenic diet was due to fluid restriction, which was once a normal part of this diet for epilepsy, and is no longer recommended. Now, when the diet is followed properly and the child takes in plenty of fluids, constipation is no longer a major problem.

More recently, low carbohydrate diets for weight loss have been talked about since 1958. There have been several advocates of the low carb, high fat diet, including Dr. Richard Mackarness, who published the book *Eat Fat and Grow Slim* in 1958, Irwin Stillman and his book *The Doctor's Quick Weigh Loss Diet*, and the Austrian doctor Wolfgang Lutz, who published a book entitled (its translated English title) *Life Without Bread* in 1967. Although more popular in Europe and other countries, the idea of utilizing the low carb, high fat diet was not common in the United States until 1972, when Dr. Richard Atkins published his groundbreaking book *Dr. Atkins' Diet Revolution*. Although the diet did not catch on at first because people were unsure about the safety of such diets and the medical community did not want to accept this alternative to the traditional Western diet. There was a lot of scorn around these types of diets, and no one wanted to talk about all the positives associated with the ketogenic and other low carb diets. The Atkins diet gained much more popularity in the 1990s when more research showed its safety and efficiency in following this diet. Also, Atkins released an updated version of his diet book at this time, *Dr. Atkins' New Diet Revolution*, and the popularity of high fat, low carb diets exploded. Other diets that were released in the 1970s (before this explosion) were, the Paleolithic diet created by Walter Voegtlin and the Scarsdale diet, advocated for by Herman Tarnower.

The popularity of the high fat, low carb craze really exploded in the 1990s and the early 2000s. It was estimated during this time that as many as 18 percent of the population was on some kind of high fat, low carb diet during this time. The low carbohydrate craze of this time even affected restaurants and food makers, who noticed the change in the eating habits of the general community and a drop in their revenue if they were focused on carb heavy foods, such as the company

KrispeKremes. During this time, there was a great deal of research being done on the safety of low carb diets, and it was found to be safe and effective for weight loss. In fact, a 2014 study conducted by the National Institutes of Health (NIH), one of the most respected medical centers in the world, studied the effectiveness of weight loss diets and put head to head low carb and low fat diets. It was found that people who followed a low carb diet saw more weight loss than people who followed a low fat diet. Also of note here is that the weight lost by the low fat group was mostly muscle mass, with very little actual fat lost on the body, while those following the high fat, low carb diet lost more fat and less muscle. This is an important distinction. It is not good to lose too much muscle while keeping fat. Having muscle mass helps to burn fat, so losing muscle mass is detrimental to long-term weight loss and maintenance. Plus, fat is unhealthy to store, while muscle strength is necessary to be healthy. So, it is important to note that, because of this, a low carb, high fat diet is better for overall health and continued maintenance of the weight lost. And what good is a diet if you cannot keep off the weight you lose?

It is important here to note a few differences between these different kinds of low carb, high fat diets. Not all of them work on the principle of ketosis and they have different ideas on the amount of macronutrients (fats, carbohydrates, and protein) that should be eaten. These are two key points to where these diets differ. Atkins, for example, does force the body into ketosis in the beginning phase of the diet, but slowly adds carbs back into the diet after the initial phase of weight loss, so ketosis is not the ultimate goal. Also, Atkins is billed as a high fat, high protein, low carb diet. The Ketogenic diet, in comparison, is labeled a high fat, adequate protein, low carb diet. There are more fats and less proteins in the Ketogenic diet, as compared to Atkins. Also, in the Ketogenic diet, carbs are not reintroduced after the initial kick of weight loss. It is a lifestyle change where carbs are not part of the equation.

The other popular low carb diet is the Paleolithic diet. This diet does not try to force the body into ketosis at all, although it could happen naturally by following the diet. Instead, the purpose of the diet is to not eat anything that was not available to our ancestors in the Paleolithic era (hence, the name). This means it is not only grain free, but it is also dairy free, as dairy products were not available to our hunter/gather ancestors. In the Ketogenic diet, dairy is an important part of the diet. It is one less food group that you have to cut out, which is also helpful when trying to stick to the diet long-term. Because, in the Paleolithic diet, you cut out two entire food groups instead of one (carbs and dairy), many people find it much hard to stick to than following the Ketogenic diet, where only carbs are cut.

As you can see, low carb diets have been around since the advent of man, and have been used to treat many different disorders such as epilepsy, diabetes, high blood pressure, and as a tool for weight loss. Also, our bodies work best when not ingesting carbs because the body was not evolved to have carbs in our diets! There is a long and well-established history of the Ketogenic diet being safe and effective for many issues in life, and can become a lifestyle. The next chapter will list some of the huge list of benefits to the Ketogenic diet.

CHAPTER 3:

Benefits of the Ketogenic Diet

There are several benefits to following the Ketogenic diet. This chapter will describe some of the most important ones, one at a time. If you have any doubts about whether to try to Ketogenic diet, hopefully this chapter will persuade you to take the leap. There are so many benefits to going low carb that it is hard to imagine that you or anyone else would want to do anything differently. And this isn't just anecdotal evidence. This diet has been studied extensively and has many proven benefits to your health.

Reduced appetite: It has been shown that, when people cut out carbs from their diet, they will naturally eat more protein and more fat. Some people have viewed this as a problem, but study after study has shown, along with anecdotal evidence, that doing so means you will be less hungry. And hunger is the main reason that people give up on dieting! But when you eat more protein and fat, your body will feel fuller longer, which means you will be less likely to give up on the diet. Protein and fats take longer to digest than carbohydrates, which go right through your system. So, when you eat more of the fats and proteins, you do not get hungry as quickly, making dieting easier. And when you don't feel hungry, yet are able to eat fewer calories, you will lose weight and stick to the diet.

No Sudden Drop in Blood Sugar: Carbohydrates digest quickly, and when the body breaks them down, turns them into sugar. This releases a great deal of sugar into the blood stream in a very short time, which leads to a spike in your blood sugar. Then, once the sugars are used by the body (which happens very quickly), you will experience what is called a sugar crash. The symptoms of a sugar crash, which you are probably familiar with, include fatigue, irritability, or even the feeling of having a hangover. It makes you want to eat more carbs for fast energy to get your body going again. This means, when you eat carbs regularly, that there is a constant spike in blood sugar over the course of the day. And this spike/drop in energy causes you to eat more because you feel your energy wanes and you feel the need for a pick me up. It causes you to eat more than you normally would to keep the cycle going, and you gain weight.

On the Keto diet, this is much less of a problem because there is no spike in blood sugar. Without the influx of carbs being broken down into sugars, blood sugar stays more constant. This means your blood sugar would stay constant and you won't feel the need to eat all the time just to keep your energy up.

Reduced Blood Pressure: Several studies over the years has shown that eating a diet that is low in carbohydrates does help reduce blood pressure. Study after study has shown that low carb diets improve heart health and are an effective way to deal with high blood pressure.

Increased HDL Levels: High Density Lipoproteins (HDLs) are often referred to in the medical community as good cholesterol. What HDLs do is travel in the bloodstream and they break down the bad cholesterols as they do so these other cholesterol molecules can do no harm. A high level of HDLS in the system is good for lowering your risk of heart disease, while too little HDLs is associated with an increase in heart disease. When you eat a diet high in fats, you automatically increase your levels of HDLs in your system. These HDLs then live in your blood stream and do the good work of breaking down the cholesterol known to cause coronary blockages, heart attacks, and heart disease. This is also one of the mechanisms that help to lower blood pressure. Eating a diet high in fats can actually be good for your health!

Increased Weight Loss: There are two reasons for increased weight loss when eating on the Ketogenic diet. First, because you are able to stave off hunger for longer periods to time through the combination of eating mostly slow to digest fats and proteins, you will take in less food. This, of course, is necessary to lose weight. Simply put, the less calories that you take in, the more the body relies on its fats to burn to create energy. Plus, since you are not taking in carbs for the body to use as immediate fuel, it is forcing the body to resort to utilizing stored fats to keep you moving all day long, through the process of ketosis, which we have discussed. This two-pronged approach to weight loss means that you will lose more weight, faster, when you follow the Ketogenic diet. In fact, if you follow this diet, you should be able to lose 30 pounds in 30 days!

Reduced Triglycerides: Triglycerides are a fat that your body stores to use for energy. Although some triglycerides are important for proper functioning of the body, a high triglyceride level can lead to heart attack, stroke, and corona artery disease. Research has shown that one of the biggest contributors to high triglycerides in the body is to eat a high carbohydrate diet. This may seem counterintuitive, but it has been shown in several studies that this is how it is. Therefore, when you lower the amount of carbs that you take in, you will automatically lower the triglycerides that your body stores.

Reduced Cholesterol: Although you are eating more fat, eating on the Ketogenic diet will actually reduce your overall cholesterol levels. As already discussed, your level of HDL or good cholesterol is increased. Also, low carb, high fat diets have been proven to decrease the particle concentration of LDL (bad) cholesterol in the blood stream. It also increases the size of the LDL particles, which have been shown to be healthier than smaller particles. Lastly, the Ketogenic diet has been shown to decrease the amount of harmful VLDL cholesterol in the blood stream. Taken together, your overall cholesterol picture will improve and your cholesterol will go down. This, in turn, reduces your risk of coronary blockages and heart disease.

Reduced Belly Fat: In a typical diet, the body digests carbs, which are then converted to sugar and used for energy during the day. Because the body is using the sugar you ingest through carbohydrates, the fat that the body takes in is stored, most often in the belly area. However, on the Keto diet, you are not taking in sugars for the body to use for energy, so the body is forced to burn fat that it already has stored to equal the energy level that the carbs used to provide.

The body stores two kinds of fat: subcutaneous fat and visceral fat. Subcutaneous fat is stored under the skin throughout the body. Visceral fat, on the other hand, is stored in the abdominal region and around the vital organs of the body. It is generally referred to as belly fat. This particular kind of fat can cause inflammation in the organs and is often blamed for the increase in diabetes in people who are overweight. Storing fat around the vital organs also can cause problems with those organs, leading to many other medical issues. The beauty of the Keto diet is that the fat burning properties target this visceral fat directly, meaning that, when the body pulls from its fat stores to burn for energy, it starts by using the visceral fat surrounding the organs. This means that you will start to lose your belly fat almost immediately and become healthier more quickly.

Reduced Insulin Levels: Insulin in produced in the body's pancreas in order to process the glucose that is floating around in the blood stream. Glucose comes from carbohydrates. If there is very little or no glucose in the blood stream to process for fuel, then the body is not forced to produce insulin. When you eat a low carb diet, it will automatically reduce the levels of insulin in your body because the pancreas will not be forced to make it. Without the need for a lot of insulin, your levels will drop naturally.

Reduced Pain and Stiffness in the Joints: Many people have reported that they have decreased joint pain while on the Ketogenic diet. The reason that has been theorized (although the research is still ongoing) is that eating grains can cause inflammation in the body, including in the joints. With inflammation comes pain, and people who have a lot of inflammation in the body can see higher levels of joint pain. Also, people with different types of arthritis have higher levels of joint inflammation. Since the Ketogenic diet helps to reduce inflammation, joint pain will also be reduced.

Improved Mental Health: Recent studies have shown that eating a Ketogenic diet is actually good for the brain, and is being used to treat everything from depression to bipolar disorder, and has even helped some people with schizophrenia! The brain seems to thrive on a high fat diet, and because blood sugar is improved, there are fewer mood swings when eating this way. Several studies have shown that there is definitely a link between diet quality and a healthy brain, and have found that high fat, low carb diets do make a great difference for many people. One possible reason is that omega-3 fatty acids, a type of fat found in many types of seafood, is good for mood stabilization and for improving overall mood. Also, the diet is said to help to stabilize the neurotransmitters that control mood, such as serotonin and dopamine. Some people have even said that they feel an improvement in mood within a couple days of starting the Ketogenic diet! There is a great deal of anecdotal evidence that suggests that people who suffer from depression are especially affected by switching to a Ketogenic diet, in a positive way. They report better moods and less mood swings.

Improved Digestion: Eating a diet high in carbohydrates is often linked with digestion problems, including heart burn, indigestion, and even Irritable Bowel Syndrome (IBS). Since you are almost completely removing grains, sugars, and other carbs from your diet, your digestion should improve. The digestive system was not meant to digest a high carbohydrate diet that is so prevalent in our society. Because your digestive system will be used more in the way it was designed to, you will feel less stomach pain, have less gas and bloating, and if you have digestive issues such as IBS, they should also improve.

With all these benefits, is it any wonder that so many people are moving to a Ketogenic diet? The next chapter will answer many of the questions you may have about the   Ketogenic   diet.

CHAPTER 4:

Ketogenic FAQ

Listed here are the top ten questions people often ask about the Ketogenic diet. Hopefully the answers given will help you clarify exactly what the Ketogenic diet is and what it is not. It should also serve to answer some questions about specific issues that people may find on this diet, including changes in body, how to exercise while on this diet, and if you need to take supplements.

Where can I find low-carb recipes?

To start, this book will give you a great jumping point for easy and fast low carb recipes, which you can find later in the book. Seven breakfast, seven lunch, and seven dinner recipes are included to get you started. Once you have tried these and are looking for more, you can find low carb ideas almost anywhere! You can search the Internet for low carb recipes or go get low carb and Ketocook books. The possibilities are endless!

Is it possible to eat too much fat?

Yes, it is possible to eat too much fat on the Ketogenic diet. Just like with any type of diet, it is possible to overeat or consume way more calories than you need for the day. And since you are eating mostly fats on the

Ketogenic diet, if you are overeating, you are eating too much fat. It is a much more difficult thing to do on this diet because most people generally feel fuller faster and for longer, but overeating is still something that you need to think about. Staying within a reasonable calorie limit is important. And remember, the diet is generally 70 percent fats, 25 percent protein, and 5 percent carbs.

How much weight will I lose on the Ketogenic diet?

It is difficult to say exactly how much each person will lose on the Ketogenic diet in total. After all, it is all about how you choose to follow it. If you follow the diet completely, you will lose weight fast. The key here is to keep your carbohydrate intake between 20 and 30 net grams per day. Second, make sure to keep your calorie count at a reasonable level. Just like any diet, eating too much can stall your progress in weight loss. Even if your body is in ketosis, if you eat too many calories, your body sill start to store the extra as fuel for the future. Also, adding exercise will assist with weight loss. See the section below on exercising and the ketogenic diet. The answer to this question is you will lose the weight you want, if you follow the diet and do the work. Doing everything correctly can lead to losing thirty pounds in thirty days! If you do not follow the prescriptions, you will not lose weight. It is all up to you.

How does ketosis work?

Simply put, when the body no longer has easily utilized carbohydrates to use for energy, it moves to other nutrients to burn as fuel for the body. The body begins to use fats, both those ingested in our foods and those stored in our bodies (especially belly fat) to burn as fuel. The body converts fats to ketones in the liver, and these ketones provide the energy that you need to get through your day. When you eat less calories than the body needs and the body does not have the carbohydrates that it can easily convert to sugars for energy, it is forced to convert your fat stores into energy. Hence, weight loss is guaranteed once you are in ketosis. This is a normal process that the body has utilized for centuries to deal with times when food was lacking. If you want to check to see if you are in ketosis, you can buy Ketostix at your local pharmacy. The sticks will react to ketones in your urine and turn its color.

What are macros and should I count them?

Macro is short for macronutrients, which are the three building blocks of any diet. These include fat, protein, and carbohydrates. Remember, in the Ketogenic diet, it is best to eat 70 percent of your diet as fats, 25 percent as protein, and 5 percent as carbohydrates. Many people do, in fact, keep count of what they eat, or use a food diary to track this. Study after study has shown that people are not very accurate with what they ate when they do not keep track of it. They may think that they are eating healthy, or of a particular diet, when they are not. You don't have to be completely accurate in your percentages (a couple percent in either direction isn't going to hurt), but it does help to keep track of how much of each macronutrient you are eating. Many people have found that food tracking apps can be very helpful in keeping track of the foods they eat and how many of each macronutrient they have taken in. There are several available that are free to use and allow you to track your macronutrients accurately.

What foods can I eat?

On the Ketogenic diet, you should avoid most carbs. The goal is to eat between 20 and 30 grams of net carbs in your diet (the total carbs minus the fiber in a food). Another thing that you should avoid is hydrogenated fats, like those found in margarine. As for what you can eat, there is a wide variety of foods that are available on the Ketogenic plan. First, make sure to get plenty of protein. You can have peanut butter, chicken, fish, shellfish, pork, beef, eggs, and even higher fat foods such as bacon and sausage. They are all a part of the Ketogenic diet. It is recommended that you eat organic, grass-fed meats whenever possible.

When it comes to vegetables, dark, leafy greens are best, as are any vegetables with a low carbohydrate content. Avoid vegetables with a high carb count, such as potatoes. Here are some low carb vegetables that you can eat and their net carb values. This will give you an idea of some good vegetables to keep in your diet:

½ cup raw spinach has .1g net carbs
½ cup bokchoy has .2g net carbs
½ cup romaine lettuce has .2g net carbs
½ cup broccoli has .8g net carbs
½ cup steamed cauliflower has .9g net carbs, while the same amount of raw cauliflower has 1.4g net carbs
½ cup of raw cabbage has 1.1g net carbs
½ cup Collard greens has 2g net carbs
½ cup green beans has 2.9g net carbs

Remember, keeping some fiber in your diet is essential, especially if you are suffering from constipation, which some people do experience when they first start on the Ketogenic diet (see below). This fiber is best gotten through high fiber, low net carb vegetables.

Also, dairy is highly recommended when eating the Ketogenic diet. We recommend that you use raw, organic dairy products if at all possible. Other options include nuts and seeds, which have plenty of good fats and are very filling. Plus, they make great, easy snacks.

To drinks, it is best to stick to water, coffee and tea.

Remember, the goal is to eat between 20 and 30 grams of net carbs a day. Your diet should be 70 percent fat, 25 percent protein, and 5 percent carbohydrates. The best place to get your carbs from is vegetables, nuts, and dairy products.

On the ketogenic diet, you should avoid all wheat products, such as breads, pasta, and cereal, starchy foods, such as potatoes, beans, and legumes, and any types of fruit.

Can I drink alcohol on this diet?

Alcohol is not forbidden on the keto diet, but you must be careful. There are many hidden carbs in most alcoholic beverages, such as beer, wine, or any mixed drinks. This is because of the sugary products used to make these types of cocktails, such as sodas, fruit juice, or syrupy concoctions that give these drinks their flavor. If you want to drink, it is best to stick to clear spirits. Alcoholic beverages that have zero carbs in them include vodka, whiskey, tequila, rum, and gin. You will need to drink these liquors straight or on the rocks, rather as mixed drinks, which will use ingredients that have carbs in them. Also, avoid flavored versions of these drinks, as they will have added sugars and carbs that provide the flavor to the alcohol.

What should I do if I get constipated?

Some people do find that, when they begin the keto diet, they feel constipated. Carbs help things move through your system quickly, so this is not an uncommon occurrence, and usually your body will readjust to the dietary change in a few days or weeks. In the meantime, there are certain things that you can do to relieve constipation. It is a situation that you obviously want to deal with quickly, not only because of the discomfort constipation causes, but also, if you are constipated, you will not be able to stay in ketosis. First, make sure to drink plenty of water. Dehydration can cause constipation, so staying hydrated is essential. Second, eat more dark, leafy vegetables. The fiber contained in these foods will help move things along. These food have low net carbs, but provide the fiber that you need to help your bowels work properly. If you eat nuts, stop. It may help the situation as nuts can cause constipation. Next, try taking one tablespoon of coconut oil. It will act as a lubricant for your colon. Taking a magnesium supplement, adding pink salt to your foods, or eating chia or flax seeds may also help, as will eating fermented foods, such as kimchi, sauerkraut, or others. Lastly, try drinking coffee or tea, which will help to clean out the system. Soon you should find that your body has readjusted to the new diet and will become regular again.

How is exercise affected by the keto diet?

There are two kinds of exercise people engage in to be

considered here. The first is cardiovascular activities, which is doing things such as running, biking, hiking, or using an elliptical machine. These are exercises that get the heart pumping. Studies have shown that doing cardiovascular exercises is not impacted when someone is on the Ketogenic diet. Following the typical diet and getting enough calories should be enough even with the most vigorous cardio workouts. You don't need to do anything different if you only engage in cardio exercise.

It can become a little more complicated if someone does strength training exercises, like lifting weights. The body does need some carbohydrates to help rebuild muscles after a difficult strength training workout. Therefore, you have a couple of options to try when engaging in strength training while following the Ketogenicdiet.

The first is following a Targeted Keto Diet (TKD). Basically, you follow the keto diet, except you eat carbs right before and right after your strength training workout. This provides your body the carbs necessary to take care of your muscles, but allows you to follow the keto diet the rest of the time.

The other option is to follow the Cyclical Keto Diet (CKD). The idea behind the CKD is that you follow the regular Ketogenic diet during the week, and then on the weekend, you eat more carbs in a "carb up" phase, to give your body the opportunity to refuel your glycogen stores in the muscles of the body on a regular cycle. The theory is that, by the end of the week of working out, you will have completely depleted your muscle's stores of glycogen, and the bulk up phase over the weekend will replenish them. Most people who do this will start their carb up phase on one evening (such as Friday) and end it before bed the next day (Saturday). Always start this phase immediately after a workout, when your muscles are most likely to be glycogen depleted. Of course, you can do this on any day during the week that best fits your schedule; it doesn't have to be just on the weekend.

During the carb up phase, you should eat very little fat. This way, your body won't store any new fat, causing you to gain weight. You should eat 1 gram of protein per pound of body weight and 10-12 grams of carbs for each kilogram of body weight during this time.

By choosing one of these two options, you can still engage in weight training while eating on this diet without losing any ground in your dieting or your training. It is important, as in any diet or weight loss system, to engage in some kind of regular exercise. We will talk more about this in the chapter on tips for making the Ketogenic diet work for you.

What supplements should I take?

Although you should get most of the nutrients you need from the food you eat on the keto diet, some people find that t they feel a little strange at the beginning of it. Suffering from cramps has been one of the biggest complaints. If you experience any symptoms or just don't feel that you are getting enough of the common nutrients, it can help to add a supplement. Ones that are commonly used that help people feel better include a multivitamin (either geared toward men or women), magnesium, a B-complex vitamin, vitamin D, and potassium.

CHAPTER 5:

Tips and Tricks to Maximize Your Dieting Success through Ketogenic

There are several things that you can do to maximize your success on the Ketogenic diet. Some of these things may seem self-explanatory, but they are very important for success. Some others may not be as easy to see, but need to be considered when doing this diet. If you follow these prescriptions, your success on the Ketogenic diet will come faster and be much easier for you to achieve.

Fluids: First, you need to make sure to stay hydrated on the Ketogenic diet. Although we all know about the importance of getting enough water to be healthy, it is easy to forget. And, when following the Ketogenic diet, it becomes even more important to do. It is especially important when you are first starting the diet, as your body may take a little time to adjust to the changes in your eating habits. Becoming constipated happens to some people, and having enough fluid in your diet is essential to dealing with this constipation. Without proper fluids, your bowel movements will become hard, making them much more difficult to pass. Others report feeling dizzy or light-headed, and this is something else that having enough fluid can help with. When your body is well hydrated, it can adjust to the changes in your diet much more easily.

In order to keep your body well hydrated, drink 32 ounces of water when you first wake up in the morning, and another 32 ounces by lunch time. Also, keep water with you at all times and sip it throughout the day.

Salt: The next thing that you can do is to make sure to ingest enough salts in your diet. When you reduce the level of carbs in the foods you eat, your body will naturally start to excrete more sodium through the urinary tract system. That leads to a lower balance between sodium and potassium in the body. The sodium that is lost through urination needs to be added backinto your diet. There are several things that you can do to replenish the salt in your body. You can start by adding ¼ of a teaspoon of pink salt to 16 ounces of water a couple times a day. It is better to use pink salt than common table salt because it is naturally occurring in the earth, not manufactured in a lab as common table salt is. It also contains natural elements that your body need for health. Besides adding pink salt to water, make sure to salt your foods with pink salt. This will also add some flavor to the foods you eat.

Other ways to add more salt to your diet include drinking organic broth daily, adding sea vegetables such as nori, kelp, and dulse to your diet, eating celery and cucumbers, which happen to be high in salt content but low in carbs, and eating salted seeds, such as pumpkin seeds, as a snack throughout the day.

Exercise: Third, to have the best results from the Ketogenic diet, you need to make sure to add regular exercise to your daily routine. It has been shown that regular exercise will double the levels of the protein GLUT-4 in the bloodstream. This is important because GLUT-4 pulls sugar out of the blood stream and stores it in the liver and muscles as glycogen. This helps keep the body in ketosis. The other thing that regular exercise does is to help maintain blood sugar levels, which also helps the body to enter and maintain ketosis, which is necessary for the Ketogenic diet to work. Plus, you will burn excess calories, which aids in weight loss. You should do a variety of cardio and resistance training, for both the upper and lower body. You do not have to do large amounts of exercise to have a positive effect. 15-30 minutes five or six times a day is all that is required. And it doesn't have to be high intensity. Even walking regularly will help maintain your blood sugar and keep your body in ketosis. Plus, you will burn a few extra calories when you engage in exercise, making weight loss happen even faster.

Protein: Next, make sure that you aren't eating too much protein. One of the mistakes people make when doing the Ketogenic diet is that they eat mostly protein, which is a huge mistake. When the body gets too much protein, it starts to turn the amino acids in the proteins into glucose through a process called gluconeogenesis. Of course, this is exactly what you do not want to have happen. And if you have more glucose in your bloodstream, your body will quickly fall out of ketosis, slowing down your weight loss process. The ideal amount of protein to eat is to have one gram of protein for each kilogram of body weight. So, for example, if you weigh 175 pounds, you should eat about 79 grams of protein a day. Make sure to adjust this number as you lose weight. The best way to get this protein is to space it out throughout the day over two or three meals.

MCT Oil: Another thing that you can do to help your body stay in ketosis is to add MCT oil to your diet. MCT oil is a high quality medium chain triglyceride that consists of long chains of fatty acids, which are almost immediately metabolized by the body and turned into ketones to use for energy. You can cook with this oil, add it to drinks, smoothies, and even your morning coffee, and it will help you to keep your ketone level up. Some people believe that MCT oil and coconut oil are the same, but they are not. Although many people use coconut oil to do this, MCT oil has been found to be more effective to help keep the body in ketosis.

Stress Levels: One thing that you should do for your general health, but can be especially helpful when trying to keep your body in ketosis, is to keep your stress level down. When your body is under stress, hormones such as cortisol are released into the blood stream, making it more difficult for your body to stay in ketosis. These stress hormones will raise the level of sugars in your blood stream. Under normal circumstances, this will last only a short period of time and will not really affect your body's ability to stay in ketosis. However, if you are under constant stress, this state becomes a normal part of your body's functioning, meaning sugar is released regularly into your blood stream and you will be unable to stay in ketosis, as the body will use these sugars for fuel before utilizing body fat. So, keeping your stress levels under control and reducing stress whenever possible is necessary. If you are going through a very high stress situation (such as a divorce), it may not be possible to keep yourself in ketosis, and this diet will be difficult for you. If you just need to deal with regular daily stress, there are several things that you can do.

To help control your stress levels, try meditation. Many people have found that mindfulness mediation helps to reduce stress. Some other things that people do include writing about their feelings in a journal, doing something fun on a regular basis, taking regular breaks during the work day, going on vacation, and making sure to have a regular day off at least weekly. Also, people with less stress have friends and family that they can rely on in times of need. Having a support system will help reduce your stress level. By dealing with your stress properly, you can reduce your stress level, improve your life, and it will help you to lose weight!

Sleep: Make sure that you get enough sleep! Simply put, being deprived of sleep causes your body to feel more stress, and the stress hormones will cause sugars to be released in your body. As with controlling your stress levels, getting enough sleep is essential for staying in ketosis. Most people recommend that the average person get seven to nine hours of sleep a day. Other tips to improve your sleep is to go to bed and get up at the same time every day, as this will train your body to fall asleep much more easily than if you have a varied sleep schedule. The body responds better to a sleep routine. Also, the darker the room, the better sleep you will get. People who have lights in their room do not get as good sleep as those who do not. Block out all light, do not have electronics in your room, have light blocking drapes over windows, or get and use a sleep mask to keep things dark. People who are sensitive to sound can even wear ear plugs if noise bothers you. The important thing to make sure of is that your sleep is restful.

Plan your food: One of the most important thing that you can do on the Ketogenic diet is to plan your meals. When you are changing your diet in such a drastic way, you need to think ahead to make sure that you don't fall into old habits. Making a meal plan, shopping with a list, and having ketogenic friendly snacks on hand can make the difference between success and failure on this diet. You can start with the recipes in his book to plan meals, then search online for more. There are literally thousands of recipes out there to use. They are delicious and nutritious and many of them take very little time and energy to make. Once you have gotten used to this new diet, you won't miss carbs at all! Many people find it useful to make some foods ahead of time and having them available during the week. If food is readily available, you will be less likely to want to cheat on your diet.

Make sure that when you plan your meals, you choose

lean, natural cuts of meat, hopefully grass fed and organic, to make sure that there are no unnatural chemicals in the meat. Turkey, chicken, pork, beef, lamb, duck, eggs, nuts, cheeses, and even jerkies are great to have on hand. Good snacks to have on hand include avocados and many varieties of nuts such as Brazil nuts, hazelnuts, almonds, walnuts, and macadamia nuts. Cheese can also be a good snack. Low carb vegetables are also good to have on hand, and they can include lettuce, cucumbers, celery, any leaf, green veggies, broccoli, cabbage, asparagus, tomatoes, kale, and even sauerkraut. By having a variety of foods on hand and planning ahead, you will find it much easier to stick to the diet. And once you are used to it, you will find that you do not want to go back to your old way of eating.

If you follow these recommendations, you will find that it becomes much easier to get in and to stay in ketosis, and you will lose weight much faster. Plus, you should start to feel your energy increase as you eat better, exercise more, and take care of yourself. All these things combined will help you lose weight and feel great

!

CHAPTER 6:

Quick and Easy Ketogenic Meal Plan

In this chapter, I will give you seven breakfast, seven lunch, and seven dinner recipes to get you started on the Ketogenic diet. With these recipes, you will have a great start to Ketogenic eating. They are fast and easy to make and taste delicious. These recipes will get you started on the Ketogenic diet, but know that there are so many different foods and recipes out there that you can use. Give these a try, then go explore for yourself.

BREAKFAST

Basic OopsieRolls

Manypeopleuseoopsierolls as a breadsubstitue, especially at breakfast time. Theycanbe made ahead of time andusedwhenneeded.

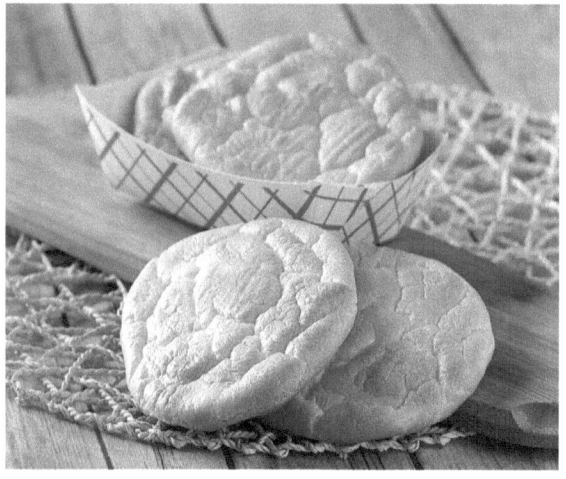

Macros per roll:

• 45 Calories

• 3.8g of Fat

- 2.3g of Protein
- 0g of Carbs

Servings Prep Time

12 rolls 20 minutes

Cook Time

35 minutes

Ingredients

3 large eggs

3 oz cream cheese

1/8 tsp cream of tartar

1/8 tsp salt

Instructions

Preheat oven to 300°F.

Begin by separating the eggs from the egg yolks. Set both in different mixing bowls.

With an electric hand mixer, start beating the egg whites until super bubbly.

Add in cream of tartar and beat until stiff peaks form.

In the egg yolk bowl, add in 3 oz. of cream cheese which has been cubed for easier beating and some salt.

Beat until the egg yolks are pale yellow and doubled in size.

Now fold the egg whites into the cream cheese mixture. Don't use the electric hand mixer here, just gently fold together.

Onto a cookie sheet lined with parchment paper, spray some oil to grease and dollop your oopsie roll batter on. You can make them as big as you like, we decided on English muffin sized dollops.

Bake for about 30-40 minutes. The tops of the oopsie rolls should be golden and firm. Let them cool on a wire rack and enjoy however you like!

Steak and Eggs

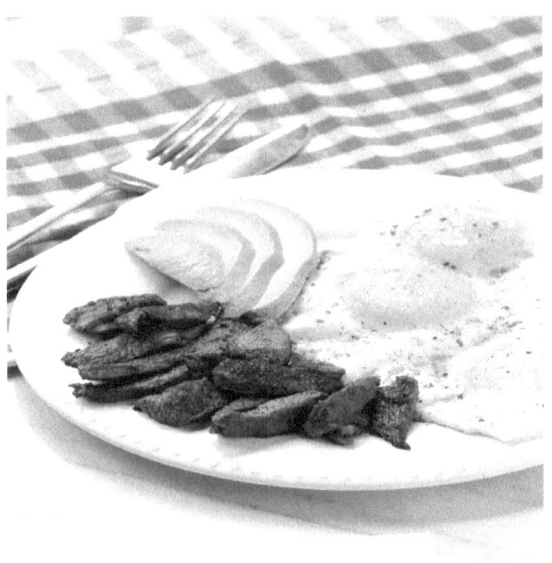

Macros per serving:

- 510 Calories

- 36g of Fat

- 44g of Protein

- 3g of Net Carbs

ServingsPrep Time

1person 10minutes

Cook Time

5minutes

Ingredients

1 tbsp butter

3 eggs

4 oz. sirloin

1/4 avocado

salt

pepper

Instructions

Melt your butter in a pan and fry 2-3 eggs until the whites are set and yolk is to desired doneness. Season with salt and pepper.

In another pan, cook your sirloin (or favorite cut of steak) until desired doneness. Then slice into bite sized strips and season with salt and pepper.

Slice up some avocado and serve together!

CaliforniaChickenOmelet

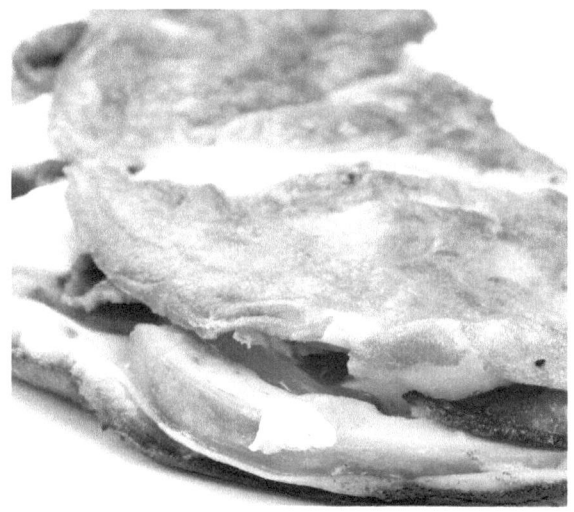

Macros per serving:

- 415 Calories

- 32g of Fat

- 25g of Protein

- 4g of Net Carbs

ServingsPrep Time

1person 10minutes

Cook Time

10 minutes

Ingredients

2 eggs

2 slices bacon (cooked and chopped)

1 oz. deli cutchicken

1/4 avocado

1 campari tomato

1 tbsp mayo

1 tsp mustard

Instructions

Crack open and beat 2 eggs in a small bowl and add them to a hot pan. Pull the sides of the eggs towards the center to cook the omelet a bit faster. Season with salt and pepper.

Once your eggs are halfway cooked (about 5 minutes), add your chicken, bacon, sliced avocado and tomato along with a tablespoon of mayo and a squirt of mustard to one half.

Fold the omelet over onto itself and cover with a lid. Cook for an additional 5 minutes.

Once the eggs are cooked and everything is warm inside, you're ready to eat. Enjoy!

Low Carb Smoothie Bowl

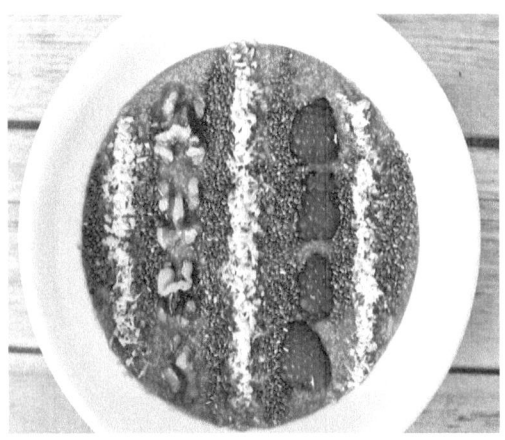

Macros per serving:

570 Calories

- 35g of Fat

- 35g of Protein

- 4g of Carbs

ServingsPrep Time

1person 5minutes

Ingredients

Smoothie Bowl Base

1 cup spinach

1/2 cup almond milk

2 tbsp heavy cream

1 tbsp coconut oil

1 scoop low carb protein powder

2 ice cubes

Toppings

4 raspberries

4 walnuts

1 tbsp shredded coconut

1 tsp chia seeds

Instructions

Begin by placing a cup of spinach into a Nutribullet or food processor and adding almond milk, cream, coconut oil and ice. Blend for a few seconds until everything is combined and an even consistency.

Pour the mixture into a bowl.

Begin arranging your toppings, or throwing them in and mixing it up.

For the sake of aesthetics, we added everything neatly to the top of the base. We used raspberries, walnuts and alternating stripes of shredded coconut and chia seeds.

Enjoy your quick and easy, low carb breakfast bowl!

Eggs Benedict a laOopsie

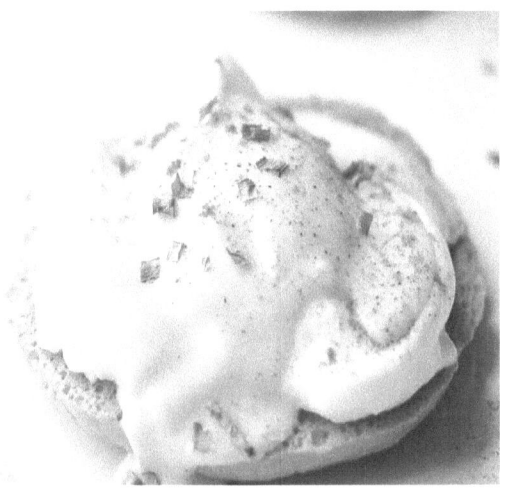

This récipe uses theOopsierecipe given above and is just one example of the great uses for the versatile bread

Macros per serving:

- 497 Calories
- 38.1g of Fat
- 30.3g of Protein
- 2.4g of Carbs

ServingsPrep Time

2 people 10 minutes

Cook Time

15 minutes

Ingredients

Eggs Benedict

4 Oopsierolls

4 eggs

4 slices Canadian bacon

1 tbsp white vinegar

1 tsp chives

Hollandaise Sauce

2 egg yolks

2 tbsp butter

1 tsp lemon juice

1 pinch salt

1 pinch paprika

Instructions

Start off making a quick hollandaise sauce. Separate 2 eggs and whisk the yolks in a glass bowl until they've doubled in volume. Add a squish of lemon juice.

Set a pot of water to boil. You need only about an inch of water set to simmer.

Begin melting some butter to later add to the sauce to emulsify.

Using a double boiler (or the glass bowl set on top of the simmering water) start to whisk the lemony egg yolks rapidly. You will see they will become thicker the more you whisk and gently heat.

Pour in the melted butter slowly all while still whisking. Be careful not to heat so much the eggs begin to cook too quick and turn into scrambled eggs!

The hollandaise sauce should be thick enough to coat the back of a spoon when lifted out.

When the hollandaise sauce is done, take it away from the heat and leave aside. Season with salt and paprika. If it cools and thickens too much, simply add a teaspoon of water and whisk to make it spoonable again.

Onto the eggs! To poach your eggs, set a pot of water to boil. About 3 inches of water here.

Once the water comes to a boil, reduce it to simmer and add some salt and a tablespoon on white vinegar.

Create a whirlpool in the water with a wooden spoon by stirring around a few times in one direction.

Crack an egg into a teacup and gently lower into the whirlpool you've created. Don't drop the egg in, rather lower the cup into the water and let it out.

Let the egg cook for about 2-4 minutes. You want these eggs to be pretty runny.

Lift the egg gently with a spatula and let it rest on a paper towel lined plate. Do the same with the rest of the eggs.

Fry up the Canadian bacon if you'd like. We like it a little crispy and warm.

Top 4 oopsie rolls with the Canadian bacon and gently place a poached egg onto each slice of bacon.

Spoon about a tablespoon of hollandaise sauce onto each poached eggs and top with some salt and pepper and chopped chives. Enjoy right away!

Spicy Shrimp Omelet

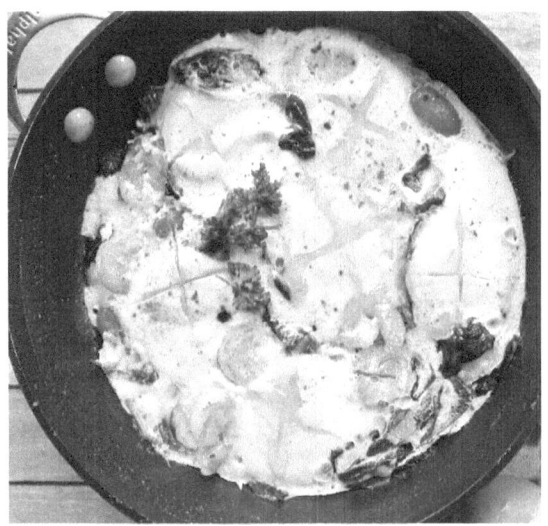

Macros per serving:

- 329 Calories

- 17g of Fat

- 36g of Protein

- 4g of Carbs

ServingsPrep Time

2people 5minutes

Cook Time

5minutes

Ingredients

10 large shrimp

6 eggs

4 grapetomatoes

1 handful spinach

1/4 onion

1 tbspsriracha salt

1 sprigparsley

1/4 tsp cayenne

Instructions

Chop up some onion and slice the grape tomatoes in half lengthwise.

Fire up a pan to medium heat and throw on the onions and some salt to cook. At the same time, place the grape tomatoes cut side down to roast a little.

When the onions are translucent throw in your spinach and let it wilt and shrink enough for some shrimp to fit in.

Throw in the shrimp and move on to the eggs!

Here you have some flexibility: you can make a scramble (on low heat and stirring very often), or you can whisk the eggs in the bowl and pour it over to make a regular omelet. We decided to make a sunny side up omelet. You can also choose to crack the yolks after they're on the shrimp and spinach so you have got two layers of egg, making a nice marbled omelet.

To make the eggs our way, crack each one leaving room for all 6, or however many you're using. Then take a wooden spoon and jiggle the whites around so they grab everything underneath them a little better.

Put a lid on your pan so the top of your omelet cooks as well. We left ours on the fire for about 6-8 minutes. Watch you eggs, once a thin film of white is covering the yolks, it's ready. If you like your eggs less runny, cook it for a little longer than that.

When the omelet is done, run a knife across each yolk and let it ooze onto the entire omelet, adding new, yummy textures! Garnish with some parsley and enjoy!

Gluten-free Banana Bread

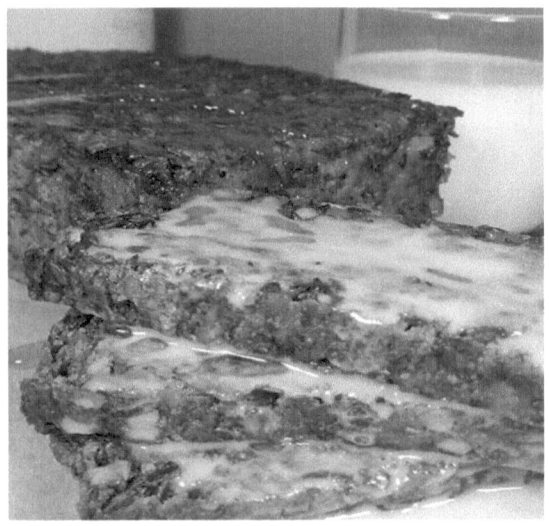

Macros per serving:

- 357 Calories

- 24g of Fat

- 8g of Protein

- 23g of Carbs

ServingsPrep Time

8people 20minutes

Cook Time

1hour

Ingredients

WetIngredients

3 bananas very ripe

1/4 cup honey

1 orange,juiced

1 pinch orange zest

2 tbsp coconut oil

1/4 tspvanilla extract

Dry Ingredients

1 1/3 cup almond flour

1/2 tsp salt

3/4 tsp cinnamon

1/8 tsp cayenne

1/2 tsp baking soda

1 tsp baking powder

1 tsp xanthan gum

Fold Ins

2 carrots grated

3/4 cup flaxseeds

3/4 cup walnuts chopped

1/4 tsp fresh ginger grated

Topping

honey

coconut butter

Instructions

Preheat oven to 410°F.

Mash up your very ripe bananas until you have a very wet, thick mush.

Take some zest from the peel of a whole orange. Then cut it in half and juice the entire thing into the mashed bananas.

Then add the coconut oil, vanilla extract and honey.

Next, add in all your dry ingredients!

Shred your carrots and ginger to fold in. Also roughly chop up your walnuts, or keep them whole if you prefer a super chunky bread. Throw all these chunky ingredients in to complete your gluten-free bread batter!

Grease a medium bread pan (about 8" x 4") with coconut oil or butter and pour your batter in. At this point you can also sprinkle some chunky sugar on top of the bread, but we like to drizzle honey at the end instead.

Bake it in the oven at 410°F for about 25 minutes and then lower the temperature to 350°F and bake for an additional 30 minutes.

To serve, let the bread cool a little bit, slice with a serrated knife into thick slices or even little cubes if you have got a lot of people over.

Our favorite way of eating this sweet gluten-free banana bread is to drizzle coconut butter and honey on each piece and sink our teeth into each dense and chunky bite! Enjoy!

LUNCH

KetoCaesar Salad

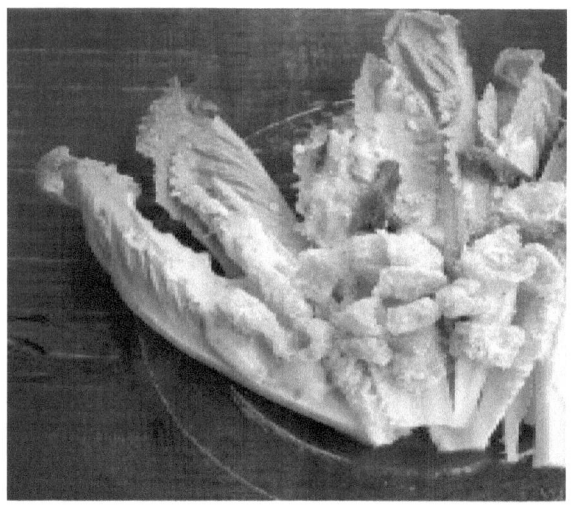

Serves: 4 servings
Serving size: 1 serving
Calories: 727
Fat: 38.75 grams
Net Carbs: 1.8 grams NET
Fiber: 0.5 grams
Protein: 13 grams
Prep time: 15 mins
Total time: 15 mins

Ingredients

1 egg yolk

8 Tbs avocado oil

3 Tbsp. Apple Cider Vinegar

1 tspDijon mustard

4 anchovyfilets

2 garlic cloves

4 Tbsp. grated parmesan

24 whole leaves of romaine hearts

2 oz. of pork rinds chopped in small pieces

4 tbs shaved parmesan for garnish

Instructions

In the cup of an immersion blender place the egg yolk, the ACV, Mustard, insert the blender stick and stand on the egg yolk and then pour the avocado oil carefully on top.

Now start the blender on low, without moving it from its position.

The egg yolk should slowly emulsify with the oil, creating a mayonnaise. (If you have problems making a mayo, use 1 teaspoon of commercial mayo as a starter together with the previous ingredients)

Once the base mayo is ready, remove the blender, and add the anchovies, garlic and grated parmesan to the cup.

Again blend on slow until all ingredients are well blended together and create a smooth mayonnaise like dressing.

Wash and dry the romaine leaves and arrange on 4 serving plates.

With a spoon drizzle the dressing on the leaves.

Divide the pork rind "croutons" between the 4 dishes.

Garnish with the shaved parmesan

Easy Buffalo Wings

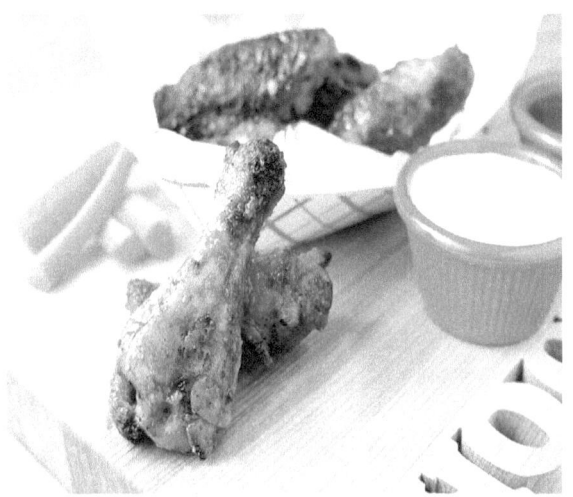

Macros per 6 wings:
- 620 Calories
- 46g of Fat
- 48g of Protein
- 1g of Net Carbs

Servings Prep Time
2people   10minutes

Cook Time
20minutes

Ingredients

6 chicken wings (6 wingettes, 6 drumettes)

1/2 cup Frank's Red Hot Sauce

2 tbsp butter

salt

pepper

garlic powder

paprika

cayenne (optional)

Instructions

Start by breaking your chicken wings into 2 pieces (the wingettes and drumettes, discarding the tips). Pour a bit of Frank's Red Hot sauce over the wings, just enough to coat them lightly.

Season your wings and toss to cover them well. Refrigerate for about an hour. If you're strapped for time, you can skip the refrigeration and move on to the next step.

Turn your broiler on to high and place the oven rack about 6 inches from the broiler. Line a baking sheet with aluminum paper. Lay out the chicken wings so they have enough space between them for the flame to reach the sides.

Let them cook under the broiler for about 8 minutes. The tops of the wings should turn a nice dark brown. Some bits may turn almost black if they're very close to the flames.

While they're broiling, melt down 2 tablespoons of butter and the rest of your hot sauce. You may season it lightly with cayenne pepper if you'd like a spicier wing, like we do! Once the butter has melted, take the sauce off the heat.

Take the wings out of the broiler and flip them. Place them back in the broiler for 6-8 minutes. Keep an eye on them!

Once they're nice and browned on all sides, place them in a deep mixing bowl and pour your prepared hot sauce over them. Toss to coat them evenly.

Enjoy them with some ketocole slaw, celery, carrots and bleu cheese!

Cheesy Bacon Wrapped Hot Dogs

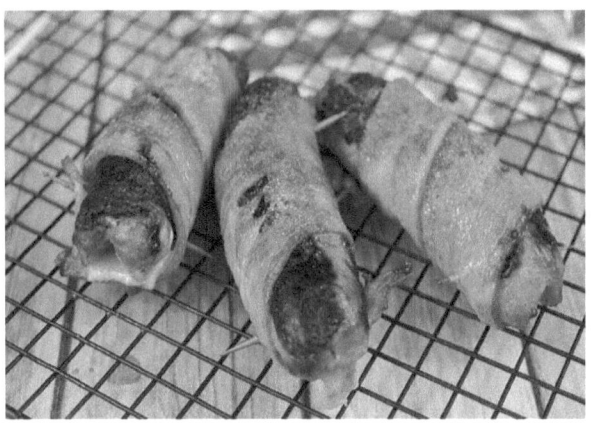

Macros for 2 hot dogs:
- 570 Calories
- 41g of Fat
- 40g of Protein
- 4g of Carbs

Servings Prep Time
4people   10minutes

Cook Time
30minutes

Ingredients
8 sausage links
8 strips bacon
16 slices pepper jack cheese
black pepper
garlic powder
onion powder
paprika

Instructions

Preheat oven to 400°F.

Cook sausage links on an oiled pan or a grill until they're just almost done. Take them off the heat and let them cool until you can handle them.

Cut a slit in the middle until the dogs are butterflied. The deeper you cut, the more cheese you can fit!

Take 2 slices of cheese and place them into the middle of each dog. If you're having trouble fitting the second slice, cut another slit!

Wrap each dog tightly in bacon. Secure with wet toothpicks to make sure the bacon doesn't shrivel and open up the dog.

Sprinkle with your spices and bake until the bacon is crispy (about 15-20 minutes). We like to flip halfway through.

Enjoy with salsa or hot sauce at your next BBQ!

Cucumber Sushi

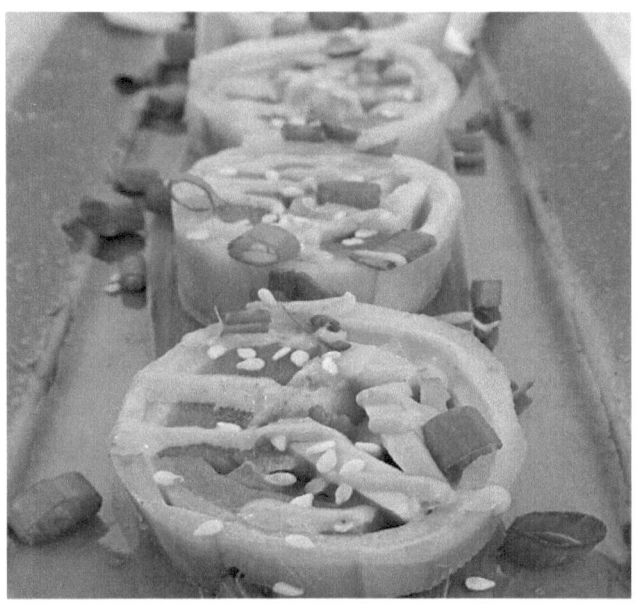

Macros per roll:
- 322 Calories
- 17g of Fat
- 36g of Protein
- 2.5g of Carbs

ServingsPrep Time
2rolls   30minutes

Ingredients

2 cucumbers

1/2 lbs. tuna steak

8 shrimp

1/2 avocado

2 tbsp mayonnaise

2 tspsriracha

1 stalk green onion

1/2 tsp sesame seeds

Instructions

This recipe is for two rolls! Start by peeling your cucumber and cutting the ends off so you have a cylindrical shape of about 6-8 inches in length.

Using a long, wet and sharp knife, lay the edge of it against the edge of the cucumber and begin to cut into it. The knife should be just visible under the transparent cucumber. We watched this video to learn the technique.

Once you cucumber is cut up to the seeds, you're ready to fill it with your toppings.

We added sliced, raw tuna to one end of the cucumber as well as shrimp covered in zesty lime spicy mayo from the night before! We also added sliced avocado. We made two rolls here, the ingredients listed are for both of them!

You're ready to roll! Take the end of the cucumber with your fish and start rolling it onto itself. Keep the roll tight so that there are no air pockets, you want the ingredients to stick to one another, or otherwise they will fall right out with sliced.

When you're almost done rolling and have about 2-3 inches left of cucumber, spread some spicy mayo on the cucumber and finish the roll. The mayo will act as glue to keep the cucumber sealed.

Now, carefully slice the cucumber into ½ inch to 1 inch rounds. It's helpful to hold both sides of the cucumber as you're slicing to maintain its shape.

Now you should have 6-8 pieces of sushi per roll.

We chopped up some green onion and sprinkled it over the pieces, as well as sesame seeds and lots of spicy mayo (simply mix 2 tbsp of mayonnaise and 2 tspsriracha! If you don't have a squeeze bottle, you can also dip the pieces into the spicy mayo).

Enjoy your sushi!

Low Carb Pizza

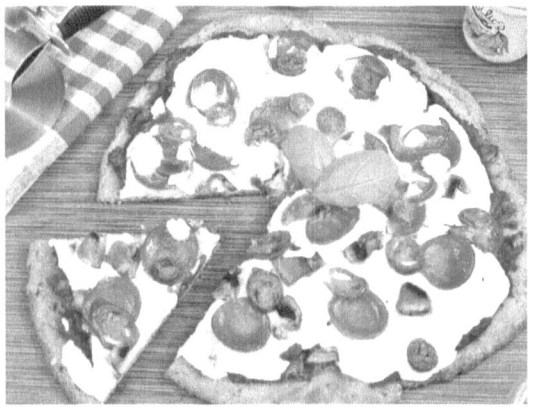

Makes a 12" pizza with 6 slices (2 slices per serving).

Macros per 2 slices:
- 578 Calories
- 42g of Fat
- 30g of Protein
- 13g of Carbs

Macros for the whole crust:
- 632 Calories
- 43g of Fat
- 42.5g of Protein
- 11.25g of Carbs

ServingsPrep Time

6slices   20minutes

Cook Time
25minutes

Ingredients

Low Carb Pizza Crust
4 tbsp almond flour
3 tbsp coconut flour
1 1/4 cup mozzarella cheese shredded
1 egg
1 tsp salt
1/2 tsp fennel seed
1 tsp oregano
1 tsp crushed red pepper
1/2 tsp garlic powder

Pizza Toppings

1/2 cup pizza sauce
6 ounces fresh mozzarella sliced
3 tbsp ricotta cheese
2 tbsp sliced jalapeños

Instructions

Low Carb Pizza Crust

Preheat oven to 400° degrees.

Melt shredded cheese in toaster oven or microwave until soft and malleable.

Add almond flour, coconut flour and egg to your melted cheese and combine. Make sure all ingredients are well combined (heat for 10 seconds again if necessary).

Place the dough between 2 sheets of parchment paper and roll into your desired shape (we chose round!).

Bake at 400° for 12-15 minutes (until slightly golden).

Pizza Toppings

Evenly spread the sauce over the crust. Get it as close to the edges as you like!

Lay out the sliced mozzarella over the sauce. Add little globs of ricotta all around (so you get some in every slice). Place all your other favorite toppings and bake the pizza in the oven for about 10 minutes at 400° until the mozzarella is fully melted (you can also let it bake until cheese is lightly golden).

Easy Beef Stew

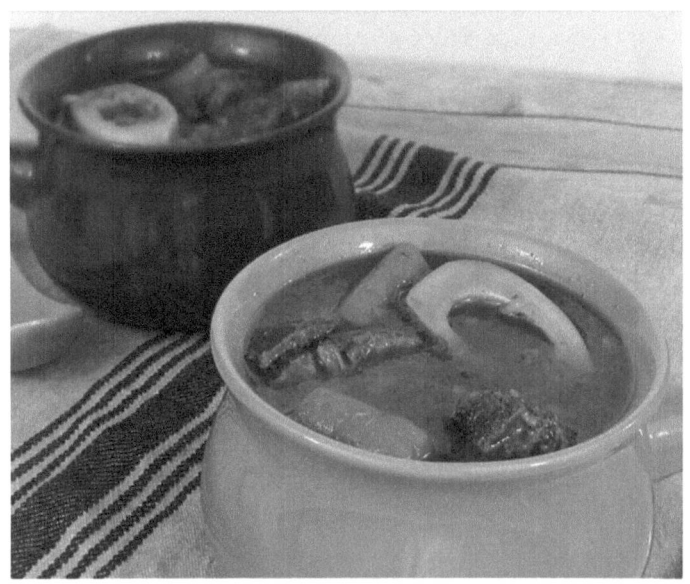

Macros per serving:
- 531 Calories
- 22g of Fat
- 68g of Protein
- 9g of Carbs

ServingsPrep Time
6servings   20min

Ingredients
5 lbs. beef shank
3 medium carrots
8 campari tomatoes
2 medium onions
8 cloves garlic
1 quart chicken broth
2 cups water
1/4 cup tomato sauce

2 tbsp apple cider vinegar
Spices
4 tsp salt
3 tsp crushed red pepper
3 whole bay leaves
2 tsp basil
2 tsp parsley
2 tsp onion powder
2 tsp garlic powder
2 tsp black pepper
1 tsp cayenne

Instructions

Place a cast iron skillet on a medium flame to heat up while you chop your carrots, tomatoes, onion and garlic into very chunky pieces.

Place the onions, garlic and carrots into an oiled soup pot, or Dutch oven, to cook a little until translucent.

In the hot cast iron skillet, sear both sides of each beef shank until a deep brown crust forms. We're not cooking the beef here, just letting it develop a crust that boiling could not achieve.

Pour a quart of beef, chicken or bone broth over the onions, garlic and carrots. Add two cups of water and the apple cider vinegar to this as well. The apple cider vinegar adds some acidity to the broth which helps extract the vitamins and minerals from the bones during cooking. You can also use some lemon juice, but ACV tastes a bit milder and you won't notice it in your stew.

To this, add in your tomatoes, tomato sauce, and spices to taste. Stir well.

When all the beef shanks are seared, submerge each one into your broth and let it come to a boil.

After your beef stew comes to a boil, reduce the heat to a simmer. Let simmer slightly uncovered for at least 3 hours.

When the beef stew has simmered for a while, you'll notice most of the ingredients have broken down and the meat is tender and cooked throughout. You'll also notice the bone marrow within the bones has turned gray and very soft.

Remove the bay leaves and serve! Enjoy that delicious bone marrow!

Roasted Brussels Sprouts with Bacon

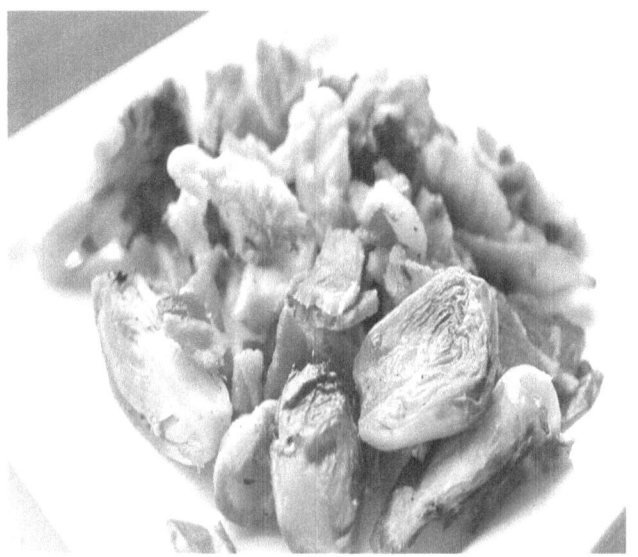

Macros per serving:
- 278 Calories
- 21g of Fat
- 15g of Protein
- 4g of Carbs

ServingsPrep Time
4people 5minutes

Cook Time
30 minutes
Ingredients
1 lbs.Brussel sprouts
2 tbsp olive oil
8 strips bacon
salt
pepper

Instructions

Preheat the oven to 375°F and cut the ends off of each Brussel sprout, it's too tough. Then cut each in half, or even in quarters if they're very big.

Throw them in a deep bowl and toss with olive oil, salt, pepper and any other spices you like. We sometimes toss them in red pepper and cumin!

Pour them out onto a greased baking sheet making sure to leave a little bit a room between them. They don't all need to be on the same side, they'll all roast up nicely even if they look messy on that sheet.

Place the baking sheet into the oven and bake for about 30 minutes. Halfway through, reach in to the oven and give the baking sheet a good shake so that the Brussel sprouts rotate a little.

While the Brussel sprouts are baking, fry up as much bacon as you'd like. We use 2 pieces for each person we're feeding.

When the bacon is cooked to your liking, chop it up into small pieces, roughly a half inch big. You want them bite sized.

When the Brussel sprouts have shriveled a bit and blackened, they're ready! Take them out of the oven and toss them in the same deep bowl with the bacon bits.

Serve onto plates and give one last sprinkle of salt! Enjoy!

DINNER

Garlicky Lebanese Chicken Thighs

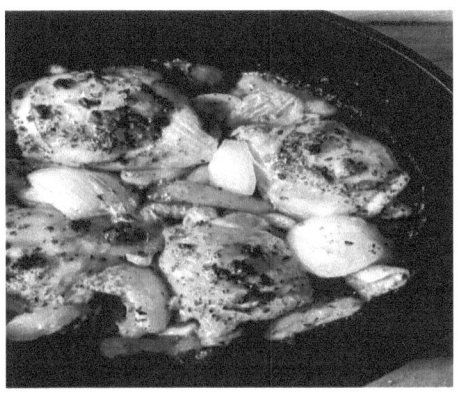

Prep Time 15 Min Cook Time 55 Min Total Time:1 Hour 10 Min

Serves 2

Ingredients

Garlic olive oil

2 tbsp ghee

4 chicken thighs

One Vidalia onion cut into quarters.

A handful of baby carrots

2 Roma tomatoes cut in half

15 whole cloves of garlic

Oregano

Juice of one fresh lemon (sift the seeds out)

Salt and pepper

Instructions

Heat the oven to 500 degrees.

Glaze the bottom of a cast-iron pan with about two teaspoons of garlic olive oil.

Add the four chicken thighs together, but try to give them space.

In between the thighs, wedge in your onions, carrots, garlic gloves and tomatoes. Add at least one or two garlic cloves on top of the thighs.

Juice the lemon over the thighs.

Drizzle more garlic oil over the top of the thighs (about two tbsp)

Drizzle the ghee over the thighs.

Generously sprinkle oregano over the dish, plus salt and pepper to taste.

Stick in the oven for 30 minutes.

Reduce heat to 350 and cook for 20 minutes until cooked to 165 degrees.

Increase oven to Broil (to crisp up the skins) and cook for five minutes or until crispy.

Remove and enjoy!

Dijon Steak and Cheese

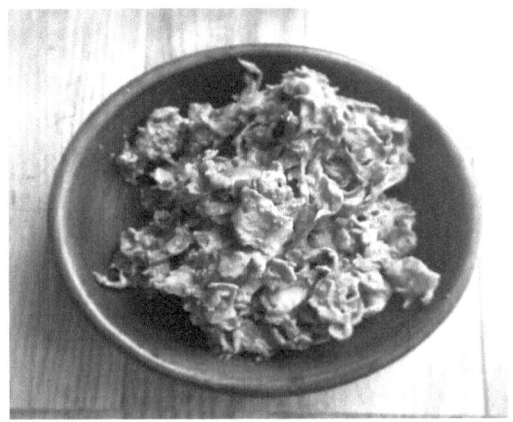

Cook Time: 15 Min

Serves 2

Ingredients

1 lbs. shaved steak

1/4 cup chopped onions

1/4 cup chopped green peppers

1 tbsp minced garlic

1 tbsp ghee

1 tbsp olive oil: I use garlic olive oil

2 tbsp mayonnaise (homemade or storebought)

1 tbspDijon mustard

4 slices American cheese

Instructions
On medium low heat, add ghee to a large frying pan.

When melted, add onions, green peppers and garlic. Cook until soft. (Frozen veggies will soften faster than fresh ones)

Add olive oil to pan until hot and then add shaved steak

Cook until browned all the way through.

Turn heat down to low.

Add mayonnaise and Dijon and mix.

Add American cheese on top of the steak and let melt for about 60 seconds.

Mix together until cheese is melted throughout.

Wicked Good Slow Cooker Pot Roast Recipe

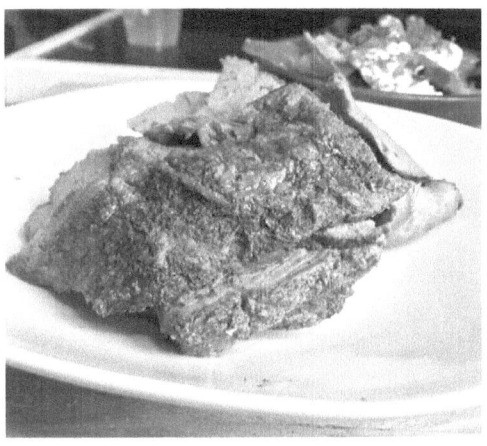

Ingredients

Pot roast (dry rub will cover up to 5-6lbs.)

2 cups beef broth or beef bone broth

1/4 tsp thyme

1/4 tsp celery salt

1 tsp basil

2 tsp dried dill Weed

2 tsp garlic powder

2 tsp pepper

1 tbsp garlic salt

1 tbsp oregano

1 tbsp powdered buttermilk

1 tbsp and 2 tsp onion powder

1 tbsp and 2 tsp dried parsley

Instructions

Combine all of your dry ingredients in a bowl

Add the pot roast and beef broth to your slow cooker.

Add 1 tbsp of dry mix per pound of pot roast. (Save the rest for next time!)

Add directly to the roast and rub it in—cake in on, it'll turn into a delicious crust!

Cook on low until the internal temperature is 160 degrees (about 2.5 hours) and let rest for 10 minutes before cutting OR let it cook on low for 8 hours until it falls apart!

Low Carb Meatballs

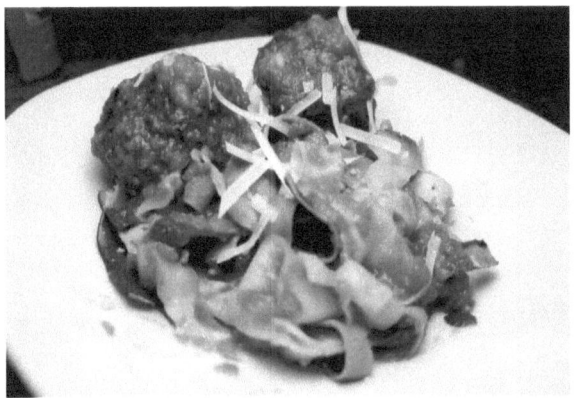

Ingredients

1 lbs. ground beef (or ½ lbs. beef, ½ lbs. pork … or … (1/2lbs. beef, ½ lbs. pork, ½ lbs. lamb)

1/2 cup grated parmesan cheese

1 tbsp minced garlic (or paste)

1/2 cup mozzarella cheese

1 tsp freshly ground pepper

Instructions

Mix it all together in a bowl and roll these babies up into meatballs. I decided to make big ones, so it made about 5 large meatballs.

You can cook them on the stove with some butter/oil/ghee but mine were pretty big so I browned them in an oven-safe pan and then put it in the oven at 400 degrees for about 20 minutes until they were cooked to 170 degrees.

One Pan Sausage Skillet

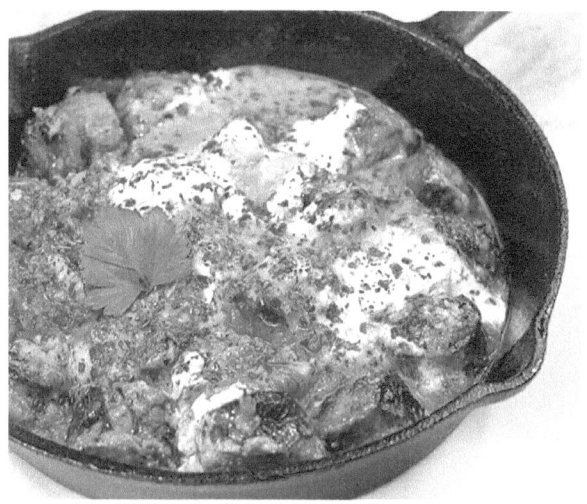

Macros per serving:

- 500 Calories

- 38g of Fat

- 30g of Protein

- 4.5g of Net Carbs

ServingsPrep Time

2people 10minutes

Cook Time

25minutes

Ingredients
3 sausage links

1 tbsp white onion

4 oz. mushrooms

1/2 cup vodka sauce

1/4 cup Parmesan cheese

1/4 cup shredded mozzarella

1/2 tsp oregano

1/2 tsp basil

1/4 tsp salt

1/4 tsp red pepper

Instructions

Preheat your oven to 350°F.

Start off setting a cast iron skillet to heat up over a medium flame. When it's almost smoking, cook your sausage links until they're almost thoroughly cooked.

While they're cooking, slice your mushrooms and onion.

When the sausages are almost done, take them out of the skillet. Throw in your onions and mushrooms for them to brown up a bit.

Cut your sausages into rounds about 1/2 inch in thickness and then add them back to the skillet. Season your sausage and veggie mixture.

Now pour in your vodka sauce and parmesan cheese. Stir to combine everything.

Place your skillet into your oven and let it cook for about 15 minutes. Once it's almost done, quickly sprinkle your mozzarella cheese so that it will melt over the top of the whole thing.

You can eat the whole thing right out of the skillet like we did, but be careful because the skillet will remain hot for quite some time. Otherwise, use a large soup spoon or a wide spatula to divide the skillet into two helpings and enjoy with a friend!

Easy Lobster Bisque

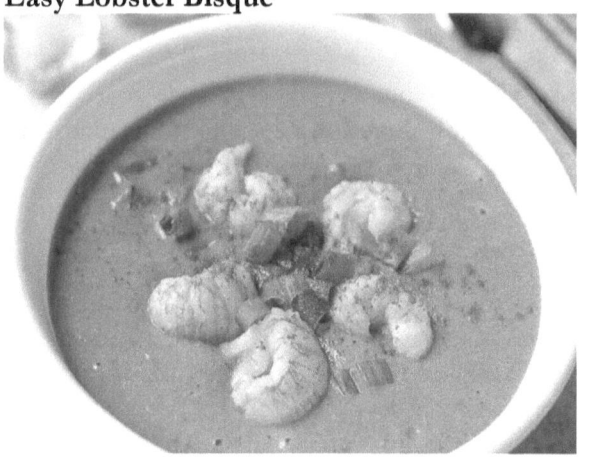

Macros per serving:

- 220 Calories

- 15g of Fat

- 12g of Protein

- 8g of Carbs

ServingsPrep Time

4people 20minutes

Cook Time

1hour

Ingredients

24 oz. lobster chunks

4 cloves garlic

1/2 red onion

2 carrots

4 stalks celery

1/2 cup tomato paste

1 quart seafood broth

2 cups white wine

1 tbsp olive oil

1 oz. brandy

1 cup heavy cream

3 bay leaves

1 tbsp salt

1 tsp peppercorns

1 tsp paprika

1 tsp thyme

1 tsp xanthan gum

1 tbsp fresh lemon juice

parsley

Instructions

Start by chopping your garlic, onion, celery and carrots

pretty finely. The end result will be blended so don't worry too much about sizes.

Cook onion in olive oil in a soup pot until fragrant, then add garlic and cook until the pan starts looking a little blackened and crusty at the bottom.

Deglaze the pot using the white wine and then add the celery and carrot.

Pour in your broth, brandy and tomato paste, stir to incorporate.

Add in your spices and let the soup simmer for an hour.

Once the soup has cooked and the spices have let out their flavors, remove and discard the bay leaves.

Add your cream and allow to come to a simmer again.

Then add in a small amount of xanthan gum at a time while stirring the soup. You should see it start to thicken.

You want to blend the soup BEFORE adding the chunks of lobster. Lobster bisque is a creamy consistent soup with chunks of lobster. If you'd like a chunkier bisque, feel free to not blend at all, but for the authentic feeling, blend first, add lobster last.

Pour the soup into a large blender and blend until creamy.

If your lobster is uncooked, simply cut it into chunks and sauté it in some butter or olive oil in a pan. If your lobster is frozen, feel free to sauté it in butter anyway!

Pour your bisque into a bowl and add your lobster chunks, stir until combined.
Dress the lobster bisque with lemon juice, green onion, chives or parsley and enjoy!

Shrimp Scampi

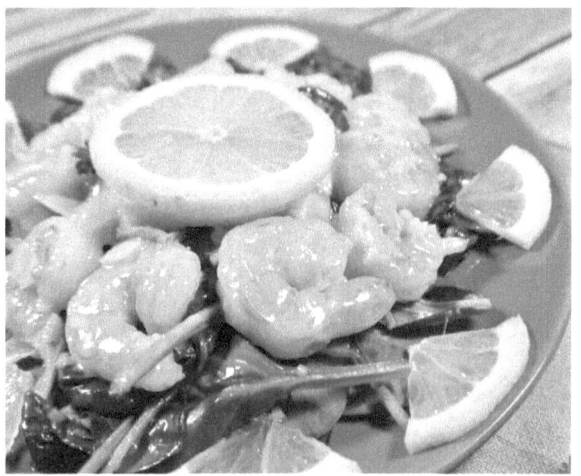

Macros per serving:

- 390 Calories

- 24g of Fat

- 36g of Protein

- 3g of Carbs

ServingsPrep Time

4people 10minutes

Cook Time

5minutes

Ingredients

40 large raw shrimp

1/2 onion

6 cloves garlic

4 tbsp butter

2 tbsp olive oil

2 tbsp heavy cream

1 tbspparmesan

4 handfuls spinach

Instructions

To start off, place your shrimp in a bowl of cold water and let them defrost. If the shrimp are not peeled, wait until they thaw and peel their shells off.

While you're waiting for the shrimp to defrost, chop up some onions into small pieces.

Pour olive oil into a pan and cook your shrimp for about 2 minutes or until they are all pink. We're not cooking the shrimp all the way through. Take the shrimp off the pan and onto a plate to rest.

Then on the same hot pan, cook your onions until translucent. Add some salt to encourage all the ingredients to let their juices out! Then squeeze the garlic and let it cook for about another minute.

Add your butter, cream and parmesan and stir until you have a combined sauce. Let this cook for about 2 minutes to let some moisture out and let the whole sauce thicken a bit.

Now add the shrimp back into the pan and stir very well. Let all the sides of the shrimp soak up the delicious sauce. Cook this all together for no longer than 2-3 minutes. Overcooked shrimp are dry, rubbery and hard to chew.
When the shrimp are done, take them off and let them relax. On the same pan yet again, cook all your spinach slightly. Don't let them shrink and get too soggy, the closer to raw, the more vitamins and minerals are spared.

Now combine the spinach and the shrimp to create one tasty quick dinner! Enjoy!

Conclusion:

By now, you should have a very good idea about how to begin taking control of your weight, your health, and your life with the Ketogenic diet. You have learned about what the Ketogenic diet is, how to get in and stay in the state of ketosis, where your body burns its own fat stores rather than sugars for energy, and what you can and cannot eat on this diet. You have seen the benefits of following a Ketogenic diet and hopefully have started on your path to better health and a happier life. Now that you have the information you need to begin, this diet can become your lifelong friend. Explore all the delicious food options available to you, plan your meals and your life, and enjoy all the benefits that the Ketogenicdiet have to offer you.

If you start today, within a week (or even less), you can be in ketosis and losing body fat. And unlike low fat diets, you will not be losing muscle mass. You will actually be losing fat to enable you to reach your weight loss goals. And with all the delicious options for food and the fact that you will never feel hungry on this diet, you will find success. If you follow the guidelines in this book completely, you will be well on your way to losing 30 pounds in 30 days! So what are you waiting for? Get started and start seeing the results in your own life!

Congratulations on being willing to make such an important change in your life. Enjoy everything that the Ketogenic can give you, including a healthier weight, improved mental health, a healthier heart, relief from heart disease and diabetes, and overall energy. You have a whole new life ahead of you!

Don't forget to grab our free weight loss report to maximize your chances of success at **flatbellyqueens.com**

YOU MAY ALSO LIKE THESE BOOKS

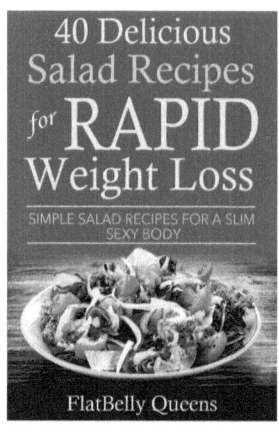

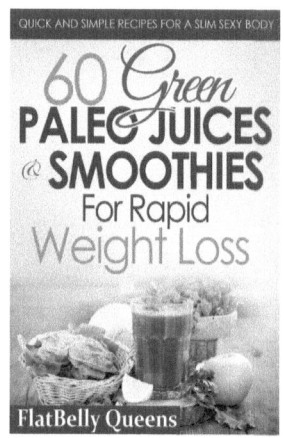

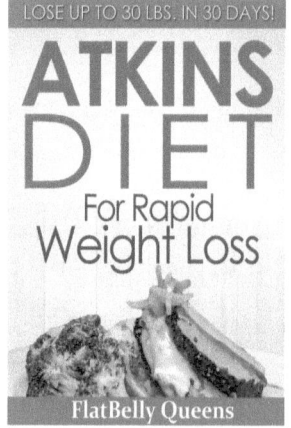

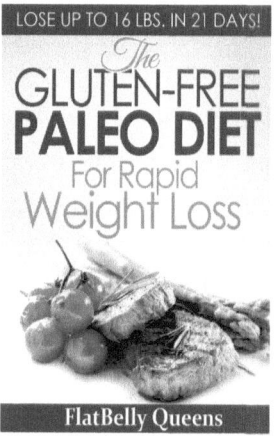